Cleft Lip Surgery

General Editor, Wolfe Surgical Atlases:
William F. Walker, DSc, ChM, FRCS (Edin. and
England), FRS (Edin.).

Single Surgical Procedures 37

A Colour Atlas of

Cleft Lip Surgery

R. J. Maneksha

FRCS(Eng), FACS(USA)

*Consulting Plastic Surgeon to the Armed
Forces of India; Honorary Plastic Surgeon
and Chief of Plastic and Reconstructive
Surgery, The Bombay Hospital Medical
Research Centre; Former Professor of
Plastic Surgery, Grant Medical College,
Bombay; Past President, Association of Plastic
Surgeons of India; Honorary
Surgeon Commodore to Armed Forces of
India*

Wolfe Medical Publications Ltd
Year Book Medical Publishers, Inc

Copyright © R.J. Maneksha, 1986
Published by Wolfe Medical Publications Ltd, 1986
Printed by W. S. Cowell Ltd, 8 Buttermarket, Ipswich,
United Kingdom
ISBN 0 7234 1057 7

This book is one of the titles in the series of
Wolfe Single Surgical Procedures, a series which
will eventually cover some 200 titles.
    If you wish to be kept informed of new
additions to the series and receive details of our
other titles, please write to
Wolfe Medical Publications Ltd, Wolfe House,
2 Conway Street, London W1P 6HE

*Distributed in Continental North and Central
America, Hawaii and Puerto Rico by* Year Book
Medical Publishers, Inc.

Library of Congress Cataloging-in-Publication Data

Maneksha, R. J. (Ruston Jams)
    A colour atlas of cleft-lip surgery.
    (Single surgical procedures series; vol. 37)
    Includes index.
    1. Harelip—Surgery—Atlases. I. Title.
II. Series: Single surgical procedures series; v. 37.
[DNLM: 1. Cleft Lip—surgery—atlases.
WV 17 M274c]   RD524.M29   1986
617'.522   86-4110
ISBN 0-8151-5753-3

**We list below a few of the other titles in print and in
preparation in the Single Surgical Procedures series. For a
comprehensive list please write.**

Published
*Parotidectomy
Traditional Meniscectomy
Inguinal Hernias & Hydroceles in Infants and Children
Surgery for Pancreatic & Associated Carcinomata
Subtotal Thyroidectomy
Anterior Resection of Rectum
Boari Bladder-Flap Procedure
Surgery for Varicose Veins
Treatment of Carpal Tunnel Syndrome
Seromyotomy for Chronic Duodenal Ulcer
Surgery for Undescended Testes
Operations on the Internal Carotid Artery
Renal Transplant
Lumbar Discography
Visceral Artery Reconstruction
Flexor Tendon Repair
Proctocolectomy
Common Operations of the Foot
Right Hemicolectomy
Extra-cranial and Intra-cranial Anastomosis
Surgery for Hirschsprung's Disease
Thyroid Lobectomy
Surgery at the Thoracic Outlet
External Fixation
Anterior Cervical Spine Fusion
Liver Transplantation
Modified Radical Mastectomy
Paratopic Transplant of Body and Tail of the Pancreas
Subdiaphragmatic Total Gastrectomy for Malignant Disease
Rupture of the Rotator Cuff
Left Hemicolectomy*

In Production
*Surgery of Lymphoedema of the Lower Limbs
Gastric Revision Operations
Plastering Techinques
Cleft Lip Surgery
Mastectomy with Immediate Reconstruction
Joint Replacement of the Hand
Periodontal Surgery*

Some Future Titles
*Biliary Enteric Anastomosis with Strictures in Common Bile
Duct
Surgical Disencumberment of the Thoracic Outlet
Aortic Endarterectomy
Axillary Dissection for Melanoma
Groin Dissection for Melanoma
Coronary Artery Bypass
Omental Transposition
Orthopaedic Hip Approaches
Management of Venous Disease
Upper Thoracic Sympathectomy
Inguinal Hernia Repair
Vascular Access
Dental Analgesia
Hiatus Hernia
Plastic and Reconstructive Surgery
Occlusion/Malocclusion
Femoral and Tibial Osteotomy
Resection of Aortic Aneurysm
Ileo-Rectal Anastomosis
Techniques of Nerve Grafting and Repair
Surgery for Dupuytren's Contracture
Athrodesis of the Ankle
Spondylolisthesis
Repair of Prolapsed Rectum
Splenectomy
Anterior Nephrectomy
Caecocystoplasty
Total Gastrectomy
Billroth 1 Gastrectomy
Billroth 2 Gastrectomy
Abdominal Incisions
Thoracotomy
Appendicectomy
Incisional Hernia
Lung Lobectomy
Lung Removal
Haemorrhoids
Rectosigmoid Resection
Surgery for Anorectal Incontinence
Visceral Vascular Occlusion
Aortofemoral Bypass
Aortoilac Disobliteration
Joint Replacement of Wrist and Hand
Operative Fixation of Fractures of the Forearm
Minor Operative Procedures
Technique of Arthroscopy of the Knee*

Contents

Foreword

A plastic surgeon who has practised cleft-lip surgery for over three decades is bound to have come across the majority of pitfalls. I consider lip repair to be living sculpture that requires the inherent artistic touch of the individual operator.

A milestone in cleft-lip surgery began in 1956 when Dr. Ralph Millard devised his operation as a young surgeon during the Korean war. Together with his mentor, Sir Harold Gillies, he published a monumental work in two volumes entitled: 'Principles and Art of Plastic Surgery'. When Sir Harold visited India in 1957 he demonstrated this operation to me, after which he told me, 'Try this method and you will not regret it'.

This book describes the manifold advantages of this technique which I have personally followed for over 25 years.

It has been aptly said that a picture is worth a thousand words and I am glad that the publisher also thinks along these lines. In the words of Sir Harold Gillies: 'The greatest improvement in the last few decades in plastic surgery is photography.'

Finally there are three types of surgeons that I meet.

The first type is the one who knows not that he knows not, he is an ignoramus, try to teach him.

The second knows not that he knows – he is foolish, enlighten him.

The third is the one who knows that he knows – he is the enlightened one, follow him.

Introduction

Cleft lip and palate constitute a major congenital anomaly of the new born. It is found in about one in eight hundred births and lists second to the more common defect of club foot. Cleft lip and palate are classified embryologically as follows by Stark and Kernahan:

1   Clefts anterior to the incisive foramen belong to the clefts of the primary palate or prepalate.

2   Those behind the foramen belong to the secondary or post palate. Kernahan and Stark's classification emphasized the embryological basis of the incisive foramen being set as the boundary marker. Clefts of the lip and premaxilla, occurring at four to seven weeks of embryonic life, were termed clefts of the primary palate. Clefts of the hard and soft palate posterior to the incisive foramen, occurring at seven to twelve weeks, were termed clefts of the secondary palate. The further description, such as left and right, complete and incomplete, was added.

Hereditary and environmental factors play an important part. A statistical analysis made by Dr. Fogh-Andersen of Denmark revealed a high incidence of hereditary disposition. As regards the environmental factors there is evidence to suggest that lack of Vitamin B_6 and folic acid during the first twelve weeks of pregnancy may cause these defects in the foetus.

The primary cleft palate may be unilateral, bilateral or rarely median. The lip may be a partial or complete cleft.

Aetiology

A century of study has eliminated superstitions and unwarranted assumptions, but a final answer is still being sought. Heredity is believed to be a definite factor, but the exact manner of this hereditary predisposition is not apparent. Perhaps the most exhaustive study of the influence of hereditary was reported by Fogh-Andersen, who in 1942 reported a study of 700 patients in Denmark with clefts of the lip or palate. In this study he discounts a genetic connection between harelip, with or without cleft palate, and cleft palate alone. Fogh-Andersen reported a 27% familial predisposition in cleft lip alone and a 41% familial predisposition in cleft lip with cleft palate. In the case of cleft palate alone he was able to demonstrate only 19% familial predisposition. Still other factors that have been incriminated are infections during the first trimester of pregnancy, nutritional deficiencies, particularly avitaminosis, and exposure to radiation.

Embryology

German anatomists Dursy and His postulated that the middle third of the face developed by a series of facial processes, *mesodermal projections,* surfaced with ectoderm that were surrounded by open spaces or clefts. Normally the processes grew until one met another, then fusion occurred. With fusion, the ectoderm at points of contact slowly disappeared, producing a solid mesodermal union. Any interruption in growth of a facial process would cause persistence of the space which was manifested as a congenital facial cleft.

Hoepke and Maurer (1938) felt that the classic theory of Dursey and His adequately explained the presence of facial clefts. Once the facial processes have met, ingrowth of mesoderm gradually elevates the depressed lines of juncture, reinforcing the union by a process of mesodermal 'merging'.

For the upper lip to develop normally, three areas of mesodermal reinforcement are needed. If one, two or more of these mesodermal masses are absent or deficient, a cleft or clefts will ensue, and the cleft or clefts will be complete or incomplete, depending upon the degree of mesodermal deficiency.

The prolabium, premaxilla and cartilaginous septum develop as a unit from the fourth to the seventh week. Obviously the term lip is not inclusive enough for all of these structures and hence the term 'primary palate' is given to this developing complex, the term 'primary' implying earlier development in the chronological sequence than the development of the hard and soft palates.

Clefts of the primary palate are due to failure of sufficient mesoderm to reinforce the epithelial primordium which will form the upper lip, anterior nasal septum and premaxilla. A true median cleft is due to absence of the central mesoderm; the central mesodermal mass may be minuscle, though not absent, producing a pseudomedian cleft. Clefts of secondary palate are due to failure of the palatal shelves to fuse. This may be occasioned by insufficient mesoderm to elevate the shelves in time to unite before the transverse growth of the skull widens the pre-existing cleft; by arrested growth, elevation and fusion of the shelves; by abnormal width of the skull; or by interposition of the tongue in an over-crowded oral cavity (micrognathia with Pierre Robin syndrome).

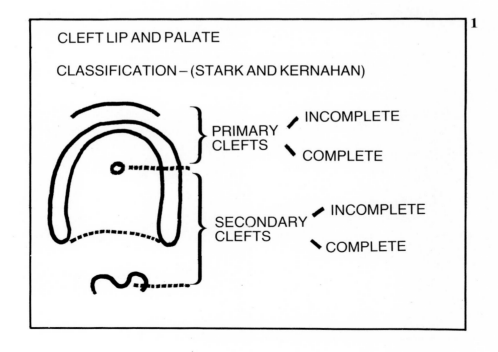

1

CLEFT LIP AND PALATE

CLASSIFICATION – (STARK AND KERNAHAN)

PRIMARY CLEFTS
  INCOMPLETE
  COMPLETE

SECONDARY CLEFTS
  INCOMPLETE
  COMPLETE

Muscles of lip

The orbicularis oris (**2**) is not a true sphincter muscle but has eight muscle components with their origins in the small muscle mass, the 'modiolus', at each angle of the mouth. The orbicularis fibres of one side end by decussating in the median line with fibres from the opposite side. The orbicularis is composed of four pars peripherales extending from the rima oris outward in an ever diminishing sheet reaching as far as the septum nasi above and the labiomental groove below on the right and left. The fibres are pierced and interlaced by the fibres of the quadratus labii superioris and inferioris and labial portions of the platysma, the so-called 'labial tractors' which pass through it to gain insertion in the fibrous tissue beneath the mucous membrane. The labial tractors greatly affect the action of this circumoral musculature. They are radially arranged as superficial and deep muscles, and most have as an attachment the modiolus at the angle of the mouth.

In the upper lip, muscles include the superficial zygomaticus major and minor, the quadratus labii superioris and the deeper levator anguli oris, which raise the lips and corner of the mouth and spread the nostrils. There is the superficial risorius, which pulls the corner of the mouth laterally, and the deep buccinator, which tenses the cheek. The fibres of these muscles insert into both the skin-mucous membrane by means of tendon extensions. Where the tendons insert in a linear fashion a crease is formed.

Cleft muscles: In the presence of a cleft (**3**), the orbicularis oris muscle fibres do not decussate transversely across the midline over the maxilla but tend to run up parallel to the cleft edges towards the base of the nose. With their integrity divided, they often contract into a disappointed, useless lump, usually evident on the cleft side. With the orbicularis oris muscle sphincter crippled by the split and no longer a worthy opponent, the antagonist tractor muscles make the most of their advantage, exerting unnatural lateral lifting and distortion of the lip elements in both incomplete and complete clefts.

Restoration of the muscle fibres with Millard's operation is most uniform and regular compared with other types of lip repair.

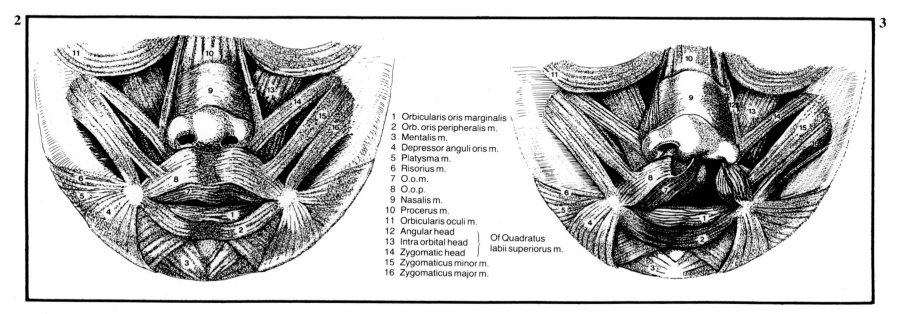

1 Orbicularis oris marginalis
2 Orb. oris peripheralis m.
3 Mentalis m.
4 Depressor anguli oris m.
5 Platysma m.
6 Risorius m.
7 O.o.m.
8 O.o.p.
9 Nasalis m.
10 Procerus m.
11 Orbicularis oculi m.
12 Angular head
13 Intra orbital head } Of Quadratus labii superiorus m.
14 Zygomatic head
15 Zygomaticus minor m.
16 Zygomaticus major m.

Blood supply

The main blood supply to the lip and nose area (**4**) comes from the facial arterial branch of the external carotid artery. The facial artery gives off inferior and superior labial branches which arise near the corner of the mouth and course as the coronary vessels close to the mucous membrane. In the upper and lower lip, the right and left labial arteries freely anastomose to form a circle surrounding the oral aperture. The facial artery proceeds upward along the nasolabial fold and at the alar gives off the lateral nasal branch and becomes the angular artery proceding up to anastomose with the dorsal nasal artery, a branch of the ophthalmic.

Although there is an interruption in the usual arcade in the upper lip in unilateral clefts, there is sufficient blood supply to both lip elements and the nose to allow surgery without slough and with the expectation of adequate healing.

1 Inferior labial a.
2 Superior labial a.
3 Ascending septal branch of superior labial a.
4 Lateral nasal a.
5 Dorsal nasal a.
6 Terminal branch of ant. ethmoidal a.
7 Angular a.
8 Facial a.

Figures 2 to 4 are based on illustrations from 'Cleft Craft' 1976, by D. Ralph Millard, published by Little, Brown and Co., Boston, and are reproduced with permission.

Anatomy of the nose

In order to deal efficiently with the nose in a cleft-lip repair it is important to have a detailed knowledge of the *surgical anatomy of the nose.*

1 Covering tissues of the nose: The skin of the nose is tightly bound to the alar cartilages. The skin and musculature are loosely attached and mobile over the lateral cartilages and nasal bones. The skin is thick and rich in sebaceous glands over the lower portion of the nose. The arteries and veins of the nose are superficial in the soft tissues; the plane of dissection in nasal operations should therefore be close to the osteo-cartilaginous framework to avoid injury of these vessels and unnecessary bleeding.

2 Lining of the nose: It consists of mucous membrane to the entire nasal cavity except the vestibule. It is thick and highly vascular. It is firmly bound to the subjacent periosteum or perichondrium.

The vestibular lining is like skin containing hair follicles and the glands at its root. It is also firmly adherent to the alar cartilages, so separation of it from the cartilage is difficult.

3 Bony framework: The osseous nose is formed by the paired nasal bones. These are joined in the midline and are supported posteriorly by the nasal spine of the frontal bone, and laterally by the frontal processes of the maxilla. The floor of the nostril is formed by the horizontal lamina of the palatine bone posteriorly and palatine process of the maxilla limited by the piriform aperture anteriorly. The naso-palatine recess is sometimes seen over the incisive canal which indicates the position of a communication which existed between the nasal and oral cavities in early intrauterine life.

4   *Cartilaginous structures.* The lateral cartilages are paired structures attached to the medial portion of the frontal process of the maxilla and the nasal bone above, and to the septal cartilage in the midline. The lateral cartilages are connected below to the alar cartilages by means of dense connective tissue, the upper edge of the alar cartilages overlapping the lower aspect of the lateral cartilage. The outer margin of the lateral cartilage is separated from the edge of the piriform aperture by fibro-areolar tissue.

The septal cartilage is a quadrangular lamina which forms the framework of the anterior-inferior portion of the septum; it protrudes in front of the piriform aperture. The anterosuperior angle of the septal cartilage is an important surgical landmark, designated the septal angle; this angle is located immediately above the alar cartilages in the area referred to as the supratip area. The major portion of the septal cartilage is firmly bound to the vomer. The lower part of the septal cartilage is mobile in this area; side to side movements are possible because of the flexible relations of the cartilage and the bony surface. The perichondrium of the wider nasal spine thus simulates a joint capsule within which lateral movements of the septal cartilage are possible. The free margin of the septal cartilage is separated from the columella by the juxtaposition of two muco-cutaneous flaps in an area known as the membranous septum. The layers of the membranous septum extend forward, diverging to join with the cutaneous covering of the medial crura, which form the cartilaginous support of the columella.

5   *Septal cartilage.* The lateral and septal cartilages do not overlap but join edge to edge. The structures are intimately connected near the nasal bones. Although there is an appearance of cartilaginous continuity, histological examination always reveals a separation between the edges; continuity of the perichondrium is frequently observed. Dense connective tissue binds the cartilaginous ends. The septal and lateral cartilages are separated by a narrow cleft which becomes obvious toward the septal cartilage. Fibroareolar tissue in this area, which is designated the internal naris, permits inward and outward movement of the lateral cartilages. The internal naris controls the amount of air that may penetrate into the nasal fossa proper.

6   *The alar cartilages:* The alar cartilages are paired structures which form the cartilaginous framework of the tip of the nose. Each cartilage consists of two portions, a medial crus and a lateral crus, which are joined at the highest point of the tip of the nose; this prominent point locates the dome of the alar cartilage. The alar cartilage after reaching the dome becomes the medial crura. They diverge as they extend downward, the maximum divergence being reached at the widened base of the columella. Although the size and shape of the alar cartilages vary, the lateral crus usually occupies little more than the medial half of the alar. The remaining portion of the alar and the border of the nostril are supported by resilient collagenous tissue arranged in densely packed longitudinal bundles.

The alar cartilage is intimately joined to the skin in the columella, the medial crus being dissected from the skin with difficulty.

The dome, point of union of the lateral and medial crura, is separated from the margin of the nostril by a triangular-shaped area known as the soft triangle.

7   *The columella:* The columella extends from the tip of the nose to the lip. The contour of the columella depends upon the shape and the degree of flare of the medial crura of the alar cartilages. The widening at the base of the columella is produced by the outward flare of the lower ends of the medial crura.

8   *Nostril sill.* It completes the rim of the nasal opening inferiorly. Continuation of the lip skin to the mucosa in the floor of the nostril has an elevation of fibro fatty tissue meeting columella medially and lateral alar rim on the lateral side.

9   *The nasal septum.* The nasal septum is a median structure which divides the nasal cavity into two lateral chambers. The septal framework is composed of bony constituents and a cartilaginous constituent, the septal cartilage. The four bony components of the osseous septum are the perpendicular plate of the ethmoid, the vomer, the medial or nasal crest of the maxilla, and the medial or nasal crest of the palatine bone.

The septal cartilage is held firmly in a groove formed by a divergence of the broad upper margins of the vomer, a paired structure formed by the fusion of the two halves of the bone.

Anatomical variations in cleft-lip defects

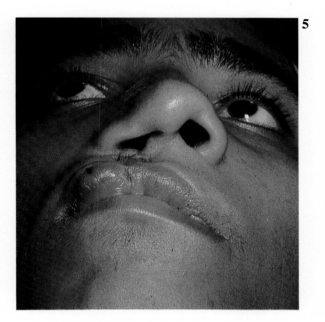

'When there is a failure in the fusion of the five components that form the nose cum lip complex during the early embryonic stage – a single or a double cleft lip results. The defect may be incomplete or of the complete variety. The degree of the cleft varies with the amount of gap in the alveolar bone. Gillies and Millard suggest that the crux of the nasal deformity is the deviated septum and the undergrown maxilla.'

McIndoe in 1938 gave a very accurate description of the deformity –

1 There is under-development of the maxilla on the cleft side (**5**) and this drags the ala of the same side, simultaneously pulling it downward and backwards laterally. Hence the ala extends as a straight linear structure from the nasal tip towards the lobule of the ear until it disappears in the cheek.

2 The medial crus of the lower alar cartilages in a normal nose are parallel and are of equal length on both sides. In the cleft lip the medial crus begins lower in the columella and is flattened as it curves into the lateral crus. This gives an appearance of the droop near the midline. Potter states that the lateral crus of the lower alar cartilage is sometimes so distorted that a ridge forms within the nostril and is sufficient to cause obstruction to breathing.

The tip of the nose on the normal side appears to be very full with an extremely large lower lateral cartilage (**6**). The tip of the nose on a cleft side is depressed and the inter-crural angle is widened. The outer part of the lateral crus instead of being delicately curved towards the base of the columella is quite flat across the cleft. The long axis of the nasal oval tends to be horizontal, while on the normal side it is vertical.

3 The upper lateral cartilage is set lower on the septum than on the normal side.

4 The lower margin of the septum is obliquely placed with its base towards the non-cleft side and often unrelated to the nasal spine. The body of the septum has either a 'C' or 'S' shaped deformity.

PATHOLOGICAL ANATOMY   **6**

1. LOWER ALAR CARTILAGE
   - MEDIAL SEGMENT – – – LOWER LEVEL
   - LATERAL SEGMENT – – FLARED
   - DOME OR APEX – – – – DEPRESSED
   - ANGLE – – – – – – – – – WIDENED

2. UPPER ALAR – – FLAT AND OBLIQUE

3. BONY PYRAMID – IRREGULAR

4. SEPTUM – – – – – C SHAPED
   - LOWER END JUTTING NORMAL SIDE

5. FLOOR OF NOSE – USUALLY WIDER

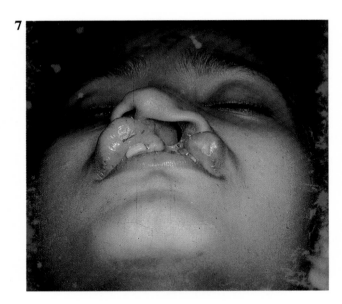

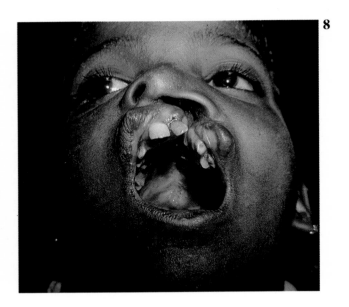

5   The inferior turbinate on the cleft side is placed at a lower level than on the non-cleft side (**7**). Very often it appears that Nature is trying to close the gap in the bony hard palate with this turbinate bone. The mucosa is often hypertrophied and vascular.

6   The mucocutaneous line of the non-cleft segment shows a perfect Cupid's bow but one that is tilted obliquely towards the floor of the nose. (The Millard operation preserves this bow intact and restores it to the horizontal position.)

7   The skin over the affected ala is often in excess and is partly responsible for the droop typically seen in a badly corrected primary or secondary cleft lip. This is the most outstanding defect of the nose in the frontal view. In an adult there may be an increase of as much as ½ inch in the total length on the deformed side. In fact, if the patient is approached from the normal side one may be presented with a prospective 'Hollywood' profile, from the other, a 'Fagin caricature'.

The role of the septal cartilage and its deformities in clefts

The septal cartilage takes support from bony septum posteriorly and from the maxillary crest inferiorly, to position the tip of the nose. Continuous edge from the nasal bones on the dorsum of the nose offers it a good profile and supports the lower lateral cartilages to form a good tip, while the caudal part helps to keep the length of columella. As the lower lateral cartilages are supported at the tip of the nose, the axis of nares is kept vertical.

Septal growth depends mainly upon heredity but many acquired diseases may produce its growth in all three dimensions. Unhampered growth produces the deformities of long nose and of hanging columella.

In the cases of unilateral cleft, deformity of septum depends upon the severity of the cleft. The three dimensional nature of the problem and the presence of cartilage in the soft tissue matrix makes understanding of the nasal deformity complicated.

Hogan describes the condition as the tilted tripod. The nasal tip is supported by the centre of the tripod, consisting of an arm for each alar and a third arm which includes the dorsal border of the septum extending to the nasal bones (**8**). When one of the foundation elements is removed the tripod tilts and alar collapses. Overlying soft tissues limit the forward thrust of the developing septum to a degree causing further deformity. There is the convexity towards the cleft side. Due to limitations on the columella by the forward thrust, it bends in a vertical direction towards the midline just posterior to the caudal border of the septum. If the tilt is severe, the septum may slip off its base in the vomer and present in the normal nostril. The vertical curve may extend past the midline and present anteriorly into the vestibule of the normal nostril, which is a common finding.

This causes decrease in the total length of the septum producing depressed tip of the nose and short columella. The medial crus of the lower lateral cartilage on the cleft side lowers while on the normal side the septal thrust pushes it further to exaggerate the deformity. In long-standing clefts, as the septal cartilage remains deformed, the further stresses produce extension of the deformities in the osseous part of the septum.

9   Rose-Thompson's method of straight line closure of cleft lip (right).

(A)   Marking the ink spots with a needle.

(B)   Measure the normal distance of Cupid's bow.

(C)   The same distance on the cleft side.

(D)   Note the 4 dot method at the mucocutaneous junction.

(E)   Infiltration with saline-adrenalin solution.

(F)   Line of incision on both sides
Note: Being an incomplete cleft, wide dissection is not necessary.

(G)   The muscle sutures are tied with knots towards mucosa. Notice the narrowing of the nostril floor.

(H)   Skin sutures from above down using 5/0 Prolene.

(I)   Mucosal area closed as a 'Z' flap.

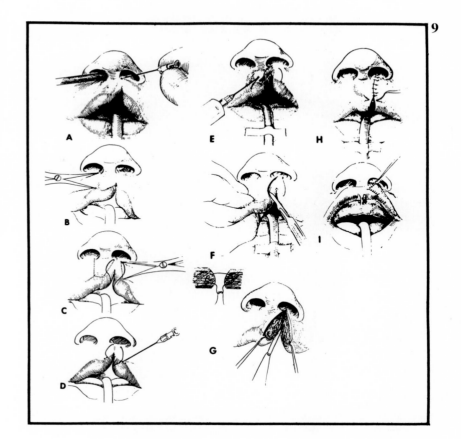

Evolution of treatment

The evolution of cleft-lip surgery is interesting. The conservative straight line closure advocated by Rose, Thompson and Kilner, later on requires minor adjustment to form a good Cupid's bow and readjustment of the nostril. Mirault's triangular flap operation modified by Brown has produced consistently good results but again *without a good Cupid's bow formation*. Le Mesurier ushered in a new era when he developed the Hagedorn principle of the quadrangular flap. Its main defect was that there was too much stretching of the upper lip in wider clefts and the nose required adjustment to bring about good symmetry. Thus the problem of cleft-lip repair was still in the melting pot – the number of cases that require re-operation is definite proof of this.

The author used the Le Mesurier method for 10 years (1946–1956) and although the family of the child was satisfied, the more I studied the results the less I liked it. There was no Cupid's bow formation and there was also a scar line running through the centre of the philtrum. Since 1956 I have used the Millard rotation-advancement flap and am completely satisfied with this method.

Dissatisfied with his own results, Millard invented a new technique which aims more at the use of the medial or 'strong' side of the lip rather than the lateral or 'weak' side. In his own words, 'both the Mirault and Hagedorn principles seem fundamentally wrong, for they take a flap from the free border of the weak side and transpose it across to the stronger non-cleft side. In principle, this borrows from Peter to pay Paul when Peter is the pauper. It was this incongruity that made me finally break from Le Mesurier'. This is the fundamental basis of this new principle.

Millard writes

'One night I had been restudying the cleft deformity in a group of Brusseau's photographs which were propped up on my orange crate drawing board. Evidently my eyes had closed for a moment and then I had fallen asleep. The bed light must have awakened me an hour or so later, and as I opened my eyes, they focused by chance on the photograph that was standing askew. The angle of its position suddenly made me aware that what we had been searching for had been there all the time! Two-thirds of the Cupid's bow, complete with tubercle, white roll of the mucocutaneous junction, one column and the dimple of the philtrum were all present but had not been accounted for previously because of their distorted position.

'To get this non-cleft component down into the correct position – that is, move what is normal into normal position – was merely a matter of releasing it from its abnormally high attachment to the columella base. The best method seemed to be a rotation incision which, while dropping the entire Cupid's bow, philtrum and dimple into normal position, would leave a triangular gap in the wake of the rotation. Thus, the main flap now became the entire non-cleft component, which had to be rotated to form two-thirds of the lip, leaving the true defect as a triangle in the upper one-third of the lip.

'The next logical move was to maintain the rotation by supplying a filler for this triangular gap. A horizontal relaxing incision on the cleft side, extended laterally just under the alar base, would allow medial advancement of the lateral lip element into the rotation gap to complete the remaining one-third Cupid's bow and lip. This advancement promised extra bonus, that of correcting the flare of the alar base. In principle it sounded promising and on paper it looked pretty good, but only by actual application could the value of the theory be proved. This required a unilateral cleft-lip patient.'

10 Millard flaps (top right).

(A) Cupid's bow marking on the non-cleft side. Incision starts on the potential height of the Cupid's bow and ascends along a line symmetrical with the philtrum and curves directly under the base of the columella. This drops the Cupid's bow component to the normal position.

(B) Millard flaps are shown with the four dot method – this helps in proper alignment of the mucocutaneous line and prevents a step deformity.

(C) The incision A advanced slightly beyond the base of the columella. This is a refinement suggested by Millard after eight years of surgery.

(D) & (E) The flaps are interdigitated and the triangular areas X and Y brought into apposition. The author feels that two flaps in the upper third of the lip repair has an added advantage over the straight line closure and prevents any delayed flaring of the nostril base. It also prevents any vertical scar contracture that is seen in a straight line closure.

(F) Trimming of the redundant tissue, this is very small, unlike the one removed in Hagedorn's quadrangular method.

(G) Closure is completed. The upper scar lines are hidden within the nostril floor, along the nostril still and in the philtrum column. Note the normal Cupid's bow that results with this method unlike the previous types of repair carried out before 1958.

(H) In a wider cleft Millard extends the X triangle beyond the base of the columella; the author has found that a much wider dissection of flap on the cleft side can achieve the same result.

11 Principles of primary repair. Free-hand marking of flaps; wider the cleft, wider the dissection – no tension on skin sutures; close anterior palate – 2 layers, pack gelfoam in dead space; pre-op orthodontia for wide clefts; over-correction of nasal floor, no dissection of alar cartilages; regular 3-monthly follow-ups; palate repair at 12-24 months; pharyngo-plasty, if required at four years, speech therapy.

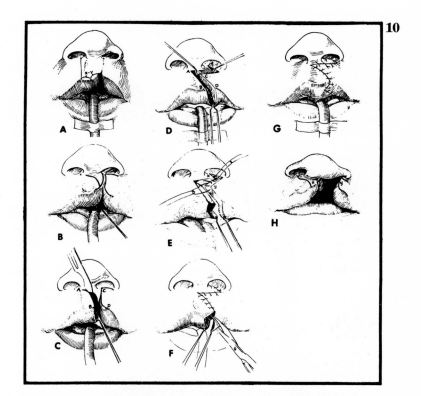

10

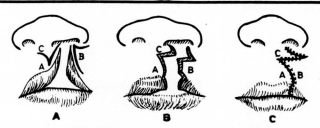

11

MILLARD OPERATION FOR COMPLETE UNILATERAL CLEFT LIP. (Complete Primary Palate.) A. MARKING OF THE FLAPS. B. DISSECTION. C. CLOSURE. Notice the formation of Cupid's bow and scar along philtrum.

17

The Millard repair

This method is essentially a 'sight' method. The normal side is not measured as in other methods. The depth and the height of the Cupid's bow is marked, and, if indistinct, calipers may help in locating the peak of the bow on the cleft side. In some cleft lips, the lateral point (where the mucocutaneous line disappears) is obvious, but in others, it is most difficult to decide. It is better to be conservative, as this line can be and frequently is lengthened.

Having visualised the Cupid's bow, place a hook on the tubercle. Mark the proposed incision line with dye markers and the vermilion border with *double blue dots*. A local anaesthetic solution is injected.

The incision starts along the medial edge of the flap, freshening the edge of the cleft, but as in all cleft repairs the perpendicular incision must extend completely through muscle and mucous membrane. This incision is continued *until the Cupid's bow is rotated downwards into normal position*. The upper end of the incision extends slightly beyond the midline.

A lateral flap is made equal to the length of medial flap. In wider clefts this carries the lateral incision down along the lateral limb of the vermilion border, past the previously marked dot. Advancement of the lateral flap rotates the alar into position.

The longitudinal incision follows and imitates a natural philtrum line. The Z-plasty above is hidden in the shadow and in the crease lines of the alar base. Note that the interdigitating is done last, and is rarely the same in any two lips. Small flaps are trimmed with fine scissors.

Tension occurs high in the lip where it is needed; the wound is splinted by the maxilla. As one proceeds in this operation, the medial side can be lengthened if necessary by extending the incision beneath the columella further toward the intact side. The lateral side can be lengthened by increasing the length of the incision toward the lateral commissure on the cleft side.

Preoperative considerations

When a child is born with a cleft-lip deformity, the psychological shock to the parents and relations is great. Some parents demand an urgent operation. It is for the family physician, paediatrician, gynaecologist, or even the plastic surgeon, to inform them that this is a curable condition but the treatment may extend over some years. The entire programme is explained to the parents, outlining the treatment necessary over a period of several years, and an optimistic view is emphasised. The parents are encouraged and placed in a frame of mind to accept the condition, and co-operate in the total rehabilitation of the child. The aim of treatment of a cleft lip and palate child is to restore the anatomical and physiological defects until the patient is able to speak well, eat well, and look well. This needs the help of many specialists, including the orthodontist, prostho-dontist, speech therapist and social welfare officer.

Surgical closure of the cleft lip is not an emergency operation. The operation is done when the child has reached about ten pounds in weight; this is usually around three months. Breast feeding is usually not possible. The child is fed in the upright position, using a feeding bottle with a large hole in the teat, a medicine dropper or a special spoon with sides elevated. Multivitaplex paediatric drops are started as a routine. Congenital heart disease may contraindicate surgery.

To anaesthetise an infant with cleft lip and palate is an extremely difficult and delicate task. With a protruding premaxilla there is often micrognathia and the visualisation of the vocal cords is difficult. Trauma to the vocal cords is to be avoided as this would lead to oedema and difficulty in breathing after the operation (for which a tracheostomy may become necessary). Sudden death may occur due to this complication.

During the operation, an unobstructed airway is maintained until the child has regained full consciousness, which should be before the child leaves the operation table.

The technique

Intratracheal intubation is used routinely. The throat is packed and the tube placed in the midline to avoid distortion of the lip. If Millard repair is decided on, the points are marked. The parts are then infiltrated with saline-adrenaline solution. If operating on an adult where nasal deformity is marked, the infiltration is made in the columella and lower third of the nose. It is advisable to wait for 5 to 10 minutes after the infiltration so that an avascular field is obtained for the operation. There are certain observations that need careful attention during the operation in a complete cleft lip:

1 The amount of freeing of the lip elements depends upon the amount of gap to be closed.

2 The lateral side of the nostril must be completely freed from the underlying bone.

3 The floor of the nose is formed by inturned flaps from the septal mucosa and mucosa lining the inferior concha. This layer is closed from behind forwards using Reverdin's needle with 3–0 plain catgut.

4 The inter-digitating triangular flaps of the Millard operation are adjusted to aim at a rolled nostril, like the one on the normal side.

5 Skin is undermined from the muscle from 2mm – and the muscle layer is closed with 3–0 plain catgut; the knot is tied away from the skin side. The skin is stitched in slight eversion.

6 A muscle stitch is put at the lowest point of the lip and at this level a Z-plasty is done in the mucosal layer. I feel that these two important steps prevent the 'Whistle' deformity (unless there is vertical contracture of the scar).

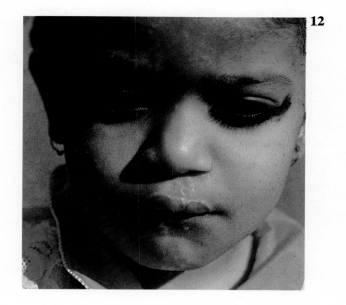

12

7 Cupid's bow: The intact Cupid's bow is present in all cases of either complete or incomplete unilateral cleft lip (**12**). Previous operations, such as the quadrangular flap techniques of Le Mesurier, failed to observe this anatomic landmark, as the centre of the bow was cut into and part of it excised. The latter method could produce a straight lip without a Cupid's bow, but sometimes it was very tight and vertically too broad.

13 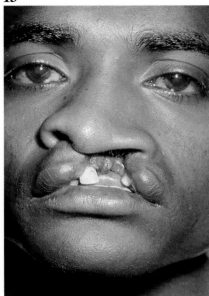 **14**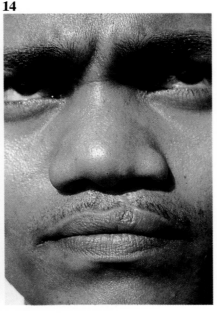

The scar in this operation runs along the philtrum. The Z-flap in the upper fourth of the lip is nearly invisible. As time passes the main lines fade and it is impossible to notice them. There is a good dimple in the centre of the lip (**13** and **14**). The arrangement of the flaps requires minimum sacrifice of tissue. In not one case of a wide cleft have we seen a tight upper lip. In this respect it is an improvement over the Le Mesurier method. It is always possible to obtain a symmetrical nostril floor. In an incomplete cleft lip an excision of a triangular wedge is required from the base of the nasal floor to narrow it and make it similar to the normal side. In a primary or pre-palate, the anterior part of the palate is closed during the primary operation and the new nasal floor is formed anteriorly by the reflected nasal mucosa from the septum, sutured to the mucosa from the lateral wall of the inferior concha. The inferior turbinate is at a lower level on the cleft side and makes the dissection difficult. As the nostril floor is built up from behind forwards it is possible to get an exactly symmetrical nostril base. We have a tendency to slightly over-correct to compensate for the delayed flare that tends to occur when there is a wide gap in a complete cleft lip. (We have now started doing bone graft to fill this gap.)

Even with the Millard operation, which usually gives an ideal lip, the nose may require further operative interference. In the very young with a wide cleft the large part of the lower alar fold tends to sag in the middle. An intercartilaginous incision is then necessary to separate the skin from the lower alar cartilage. We advance medially the lower flap of cartilage and mucosa. The rearranged flap is retained in this new position by two or three mattress sutures tied over small rubber tubes on the skin side. In adult patients the winged incision of Rethi is used to expose the affected dome of the alar cartilage. This is sometimes built up with soft tissue onlay graft (taken from the redundant flap material) or with a cartilage graft from the ear. In some cases we do a division of the medial end of the lower alar cartilage and fix it at a higher level again, with a mattress stitch tied on the skin side. We have not used wire stitches joining the two opposite alar cartilages, but it seems a good procedure. When we close the winged incision an ellipse of skin is excised from the lower skin flap on the affected side. We have found the insertion of a rubber tube into the newly formed nostril helpful in putting the cardinal stitch at the nostril base. The tube should be equal to the circumference of the normal nostril.

(A)   The lip is closed in three layers. The muscle is approximated by 3–0 catgut with the knot tied on the mucosa side.

(B)   Muscle in the most dependent part of the lip is closed similarly. This avoids any separation of the flaps and a late 'whistle' deformity.

(C)   The dependent mucosa is stitched with either a vertical or transverse mattress stitch. This prevents any infolding of the mucosa.

(D)   A Z-plasty is done in the lowest part of the lip.

After the operation a dry gauze is applied with a surgical tape cover. The operated area is left open after 36 to 48 hours. The stitches are removed on the fifth day. In young children both the elbows are fixed in extension by padded wooden splints. Sometimes the splints are joined together with another strap going behind the back of the child.

We do not apply a Logan's bow as a routine. When a very wide cleft has been closed, the bow is put on at the time of removal of the stitches and retained for 48 hours. This prevents any sudden strain on the lip and also protects the recently healed lip from accidental injury. After the stitches are removed a cold cream is advised for local application on the lip.

For post-operative sedation we use either Oblivon or Largactil in syrup form. It is important to realise that a child with a complete cleft lip is accustomed to breathing through a wide opening and with the closure of the lip there is a substantial decrease and the breathing mechanism has to adjust to this. In the early stages oxygen inhalation may be necessary and helpful until the child breathes freely on its own. The operation should be completed satisfactorily within a reasonable period of time as prolonged anaesthesia produces vasodepression. If added to this, there is any evidence of malnutrition and anaemia, a circulatory crisis could be fatal.

Patients are regularly called for follow-up. Photographs are usually taken after every six months. Follow-up cards are given and the improvement in the alveolar arch is observed. If need be, orthodontic treatment is advised.

Operative steps

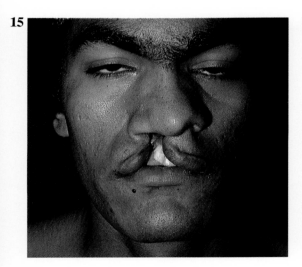

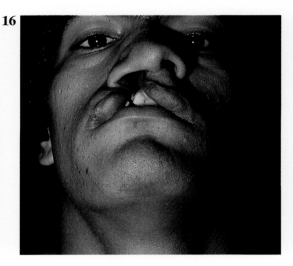

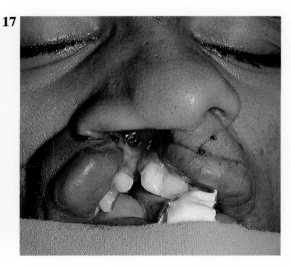

15 Primary cleft lip of the right side in an adult. Notice the flared deformity of the nostril, the intact Cupid's bow on the medial side which is tilted upwards and has to be brought down to normal position at operation. Muscle tissues are well developed. An ideal case for demonstration. Such adult clefts are often seen in Third World countries

16 Nasal view showing the wide gap in the soft tissues and bony alveolus. Notice the typical defect of the nostril with the depressed alar dome. Imagine the shape of the lower alar cartilage. The lower part of septal cartilage is protruding in the non-cleft side. The incisor tooth is rotated.

17 After intubation anaesthesia, the throat is packed (or cuff tube). The surgeon sits on the head end with an assistant on his left side. A shoulder pad is positioned and head slightly lowered and steadied on a ring. The operating distance varies with each surgeon if using magnification glasses. Notice the markings on the medial segment which will form the upper part of the interdigitating flap in the final repair. *The Cupid's bow is maintained by this marking.*

21

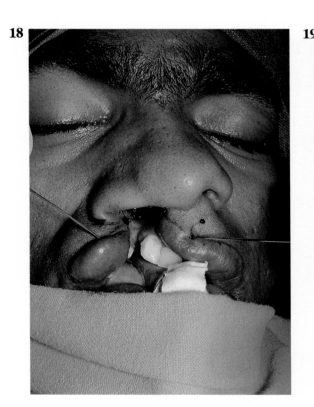

18

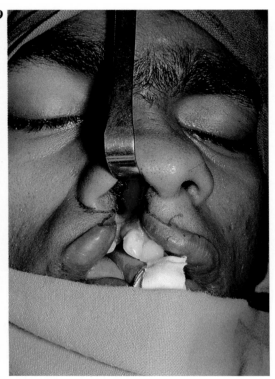

19

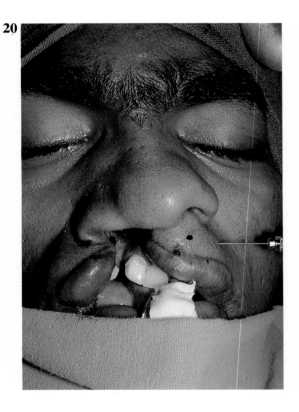

20

18 and **19** Notice the slanting lower part of the septum, the gap in the bony alveolus and the rotated incisor tooth. Markings are made on the lateral segment, the length of the upper line varies according to the width of the gap to be closed. The lower lateral point is where the lip starts to thin down. Note that calipers are unnecessary, this is a 'sight method', as well as a 'cut as you go' method. The essential points are punctured with a needle to retain the landmarks at the time of closure. *The four point method on the mucocutaneous margin helps to avoid to step defect in the final result.*

20 Tissues are ballooned out with saline-adrenalin solution. This controls bleeding and helps in proper approximation of tissues. Wait for a couple of minutes before starting the operation.

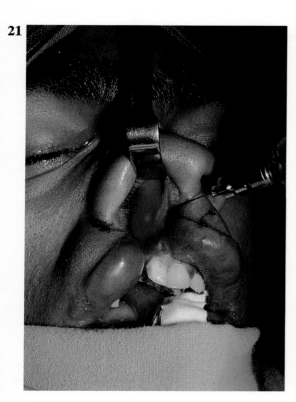

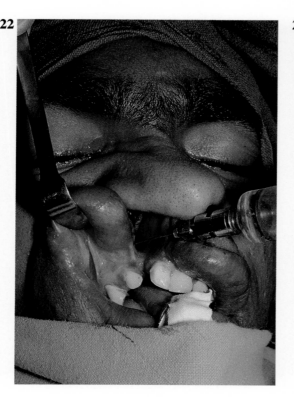

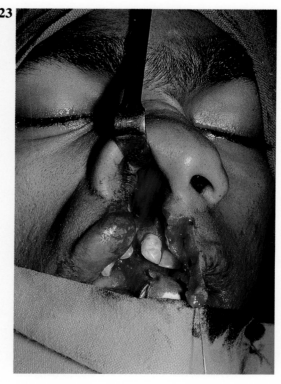

21 Infiltration of the septal mucosa. Decide on the level at which the mucosa is to be incised. The two flaps are then used to form the nasal and oral layers in closing the anterior palate extending up to the back of the primary palate, as in this case.

22 The inferior turbinate on the cleft side is usually lower than the one on the non-cleft side – the mucosa over the turbinate is infiltrated with saline-adrenaline and this infiltration is also extended to the buccal sulcus and premaxillary area.

23 Incision of the medial segment is commenced from the septal mucosa and reaches the higher point at the side of the columella. From here with a No. 11 blade the edge of the flap is pared to reach the highest point of the Cupid's bow; the incision then extends medially to a point below the base of the columella. In Millard's second procedure this is extended still further beyond the midline but the author has not found this necessary. The free end of the lip is held with a stitch and bleeding controlled. This is usually from the cut end of the superior labial artery.

24	25	26
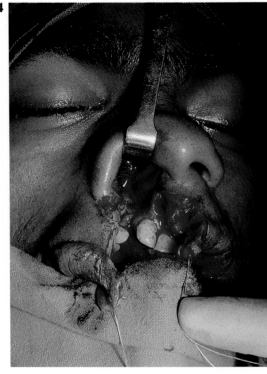	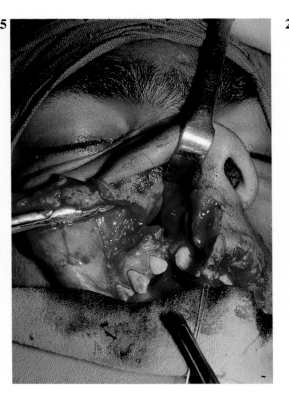	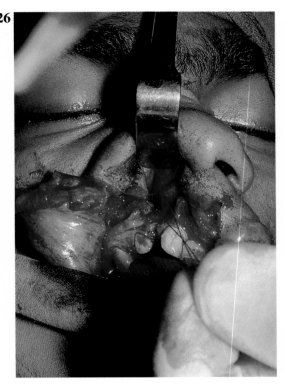

24 The lateral lip segment is then incised from above downwards and the free end is held up. Bleeding is controlled.

25 From the top point of the lateral segment the incision is carried towards the inferior turbinate. A second incision is now joined to the first to extend along the buccal sulcus – the length of this incision depends upon the gap to be closed. Through the buccal incision the soft tissue over the maxilla and the outer side of the alar cartilage is dissected free from the underlying bone. This completely dissects off the lip elements from the underlying bone and should be tested to see if it can be advanced freely towards the middle. *Inadequate dissection* is the root cause of poor result on the suture line and ultimately poor result of the cleft-lip surgery.

26 To begin the formation of the anterior palate the upper layer of the septal mucosa and the mucosa from the inferior turbinate are stitched with either 3–0 catgut or Dexon. This is a difficult stitch and needs a fully curved small needle to work in a small gap.

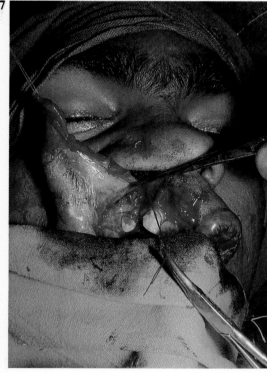

27 The stitch is held with forceps and this helps to close the oral layer.

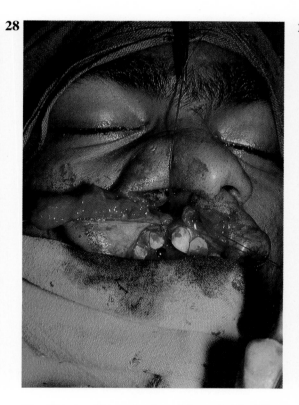

28 The oral layer is closed from behind forwards. A dead space is left between the oral and nasal layers – some surgeons fill up this area with antogenous bone grafts.

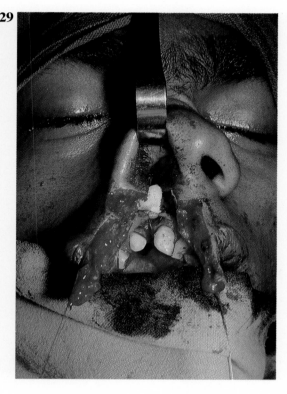

29 The gap is filled with dental gelfoam gauze – this is useful to close the dead space.

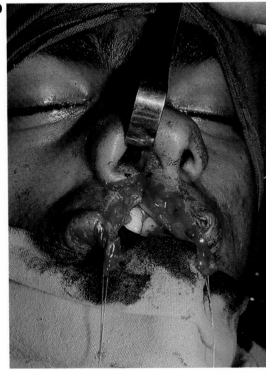

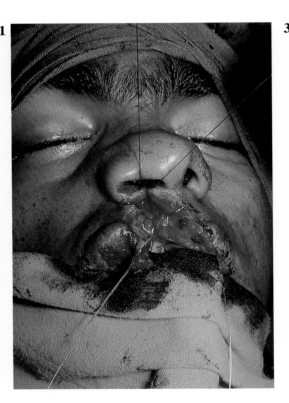

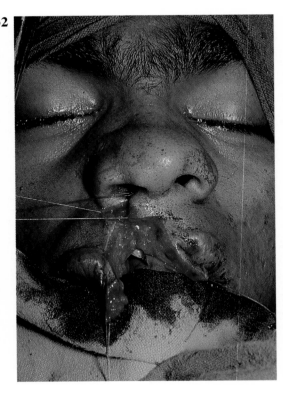

30 The closure of the anterior cleft approaches the two upper points already marked (A and B). From this stage the closure of the lip elements begin.

31 Once the two landmarks are stitched the surgeon confirms that the nostril floor is equal on both sides. In a wide cleft it is better to overcorrect the floor slightly to allow for the delayed flaring that usually occurs – taking this precaution has helped in preventing this very common deformity seen in secondary cleft defects.

32 The muscular layer of the upper third of the lip is now closed with 3–0 catgut using inverted interrupted stitches. The knot on the deeper side promotes better healing of the skin margins.

33

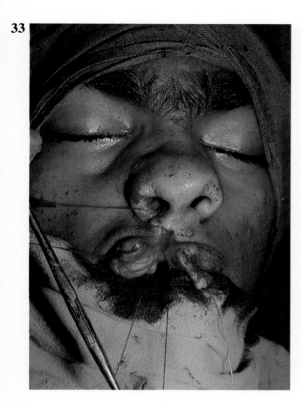

34

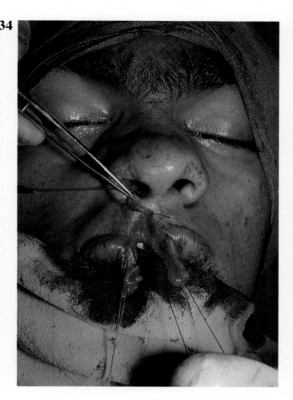

35

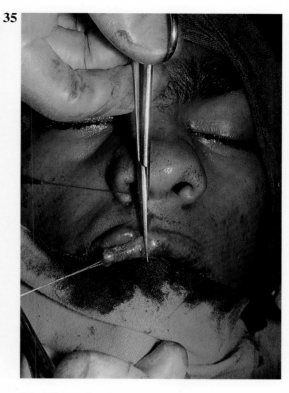

33 The mucosal layer is closed from above downwards with catgut.

34 The upper two thirds of the lip is now ready for skin closure and here either 5 or 6–0 prolene is preferred. The knots sit 'easy' on the apposed margins and thus leave no stitch marks on the skin surface. 'A surgeon is known by his stitch marks.'

35 The redundant part of the medial segment is now excised as shown, if a straight line closure is to be made in this part of the lip. There are many variants in this and a zig-zag closure is also very popular.

36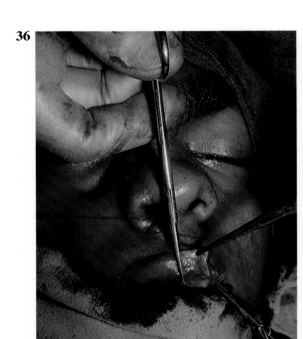

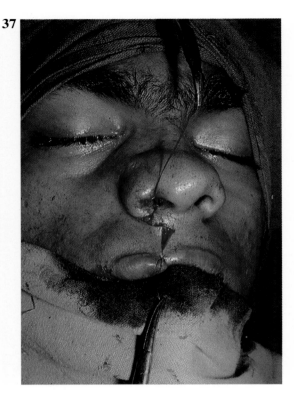

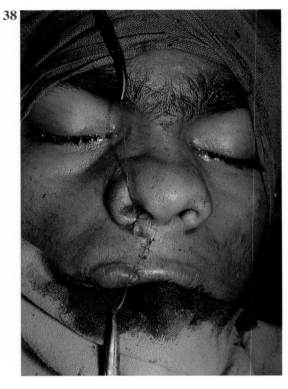

36 Similarly the redundant part of the lateral segment is excised in a straight line.

37 The mucocutaneous junction is carefully approximated and if the four dot method has been used the margin of error is much reduced. The 'white roll' method popularised by Dr. Millard seems rather difficult to carry out.

38 The remaining part of the skin is closed with fine prolene. Avoid inversion of the skin margins but rather stitch in slight eversion as this helps to form the ridge of the philtrum.

39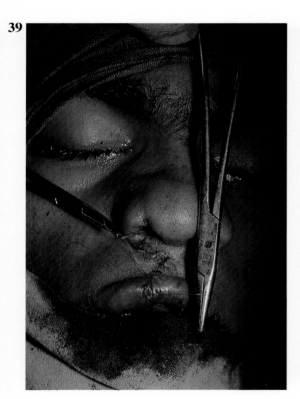

40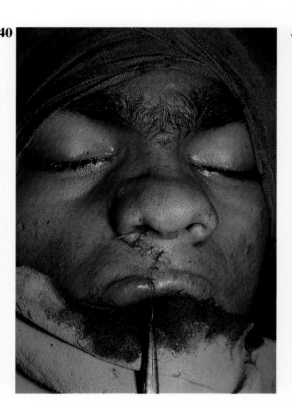

41

39 and **40**   The mucosa is closed with vertical mattress sutures using prolene. This type of stitch avoids the tendency of the mucosa to infold, unlike the skin layer. Infolding is responsible for the whistle defect in the lower part of the lip.

41   Mucosal suturing is completed.

42

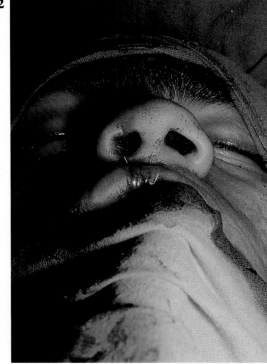

42 Nostril view to note the symmetry of both sides. It is often said that the surgeon is so enamoured with his lip result that he forgets the nostril apertures! It is at this time that any minor trimming may be ideal for a good result.

43

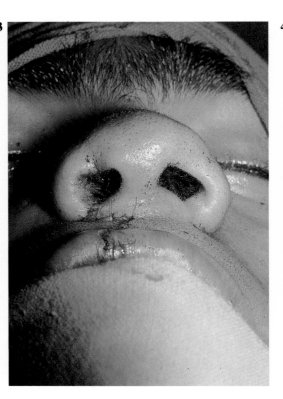

43 A much nearer view of the nostril before the dressing is applied.

44

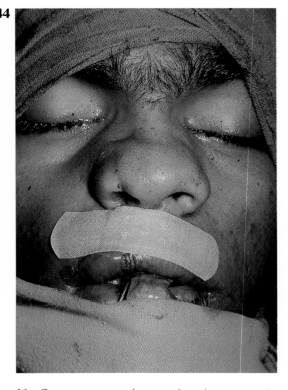

44 Some surgeons keep a dressing, some do not. Some even use Logan's bow when there is much tension on the suture line. In young children the hands are strapped with splints. Sutures are removed by the fourth or fifth day.

Notice that good alar dome symmetry has been achieved without any dissection of the alar cartilage. If the dome is still depressed the author has used muscular tissue from the redundant excised part of the lip as an 'onlay' graft. This is inserted through a midcolumellar incision rather than by Joseph's incision on the exposed part of the nose. Alar rim excisions should be undertaken with care.

Case reports

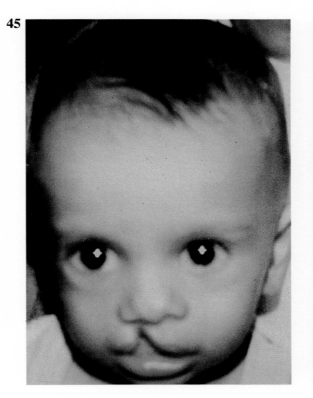
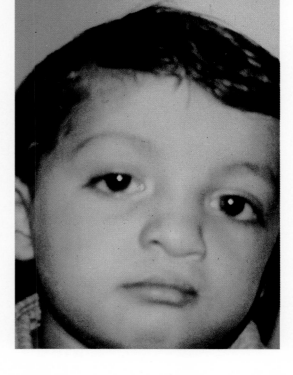

45 and **46**   **Unilateral incomplete cleft lip of
the right side.** Rotation advancement flap used
to repair the defect. Result after 10 years of
surgery with good Cupid's bow and faint scar
line (**46**). Slight muscle buckling on the lower
lateral segment.

47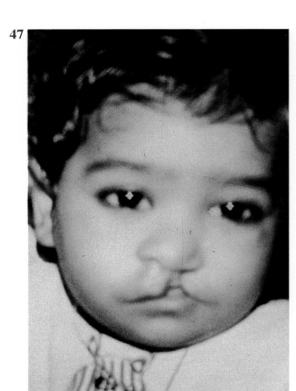

48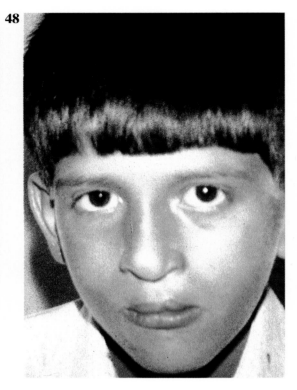

49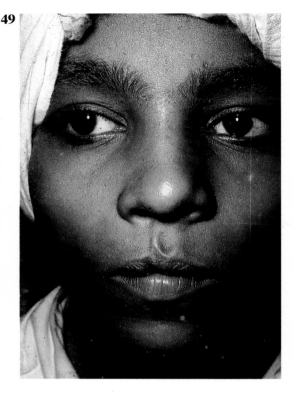

47 and **48** **Incomplete cleft** has minimal tissue missing except for a marked failure in down growth of the non-cleft dimple Cupid's bow component. This necessitates radical rotation but with minimal advancement. Natural and uninterrupted position of the dimple and Cupid's bow is the reward. The scar hidden in the semblance of a philtrum column on the cleft side seems a reasonable price to pay.

49 and **50** **Right-sided incomplete cleft.** Girl aged 14. Notice the intact Cupid's bow which is in the misplaced position with slight flaring of the nasal floor. Alar dome is uniform to start with and hence an easy repair using the advancement-rotation flap of Millard. In the postoperative result notice the dimple and the philtrum.

50

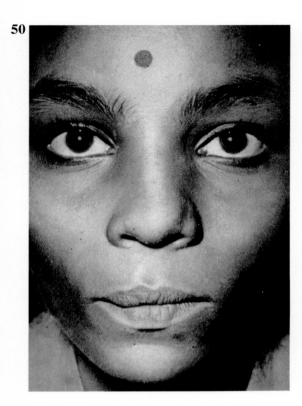

51

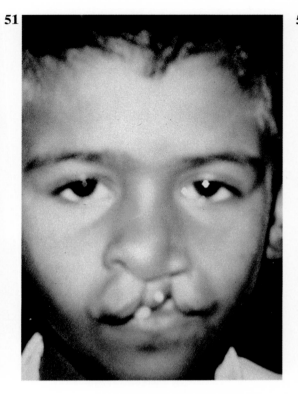

52

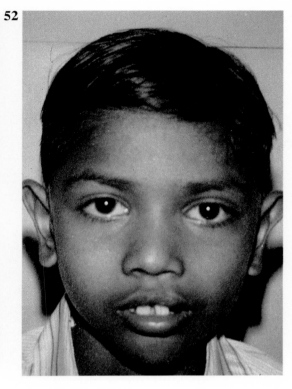

51 and **52** **Left-sided unilateral incomplete cleft.** Notice the widened nostril floor typical of this deformity. Eight years after corrective surgery, notice the faint scar and normal lip contour. No secondary correction will be needed in future. Good result.

53

54

55

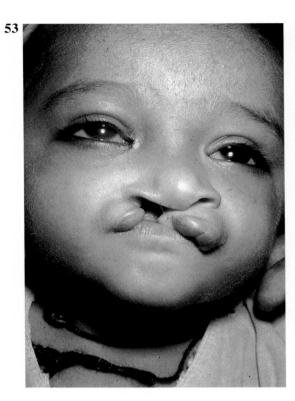

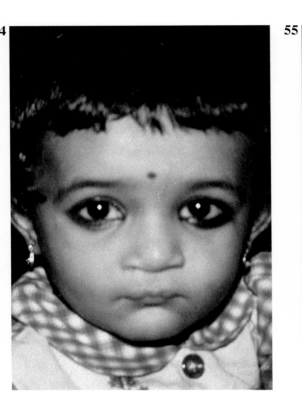

53 and **54** **Right-sided incomplete cleft in six-month-old baby.** Rotation advancement flap used to create faint scarline and Cupid's bow. Postoperative photo at 4 years (**54**).

55 and **56** **Left-sided incomplete cleft lip.** Patient returned 18 years later as an adult. Well adjusted to life with a good future ahead of her. Notice the faint scar line and good Cupid's bow – the two main advantages of Millard's repair.

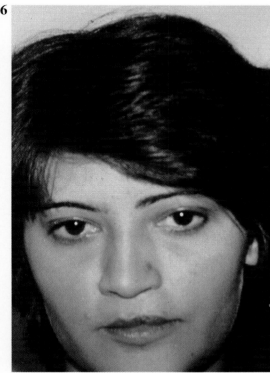

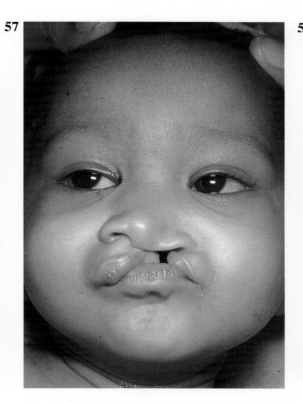

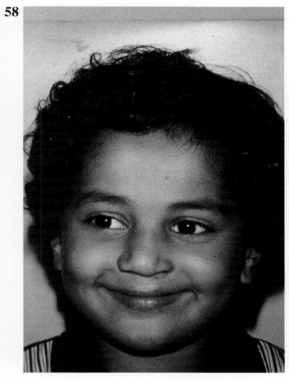

57 and **58** **Left-sided unilateral cleft.** Result after seven years. Child is well adjusted to school life and willingly posed for a picture. Notice the faint scar line and the well marked Cupid's bow to produce a good result.

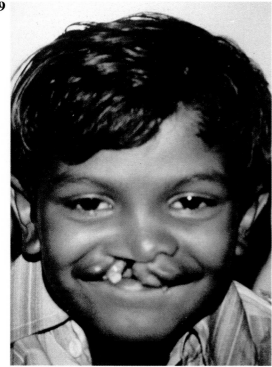 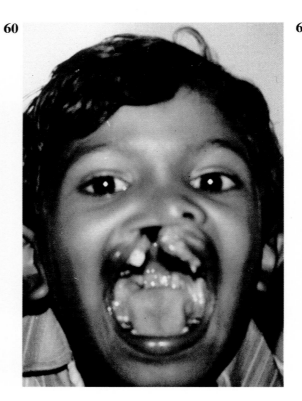 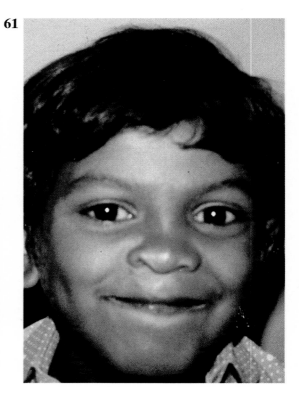

59 to **61** **Right-sided complete cleft of lip and palate with wide bony gap.** After primary closure of the palate the lip repair was undertaken in 1981. Using the advancement rotation principle the lateral lip elements were radically brought to the midline. Notice the faint scar line and good alar margin without any intranasal operative procedure.

62

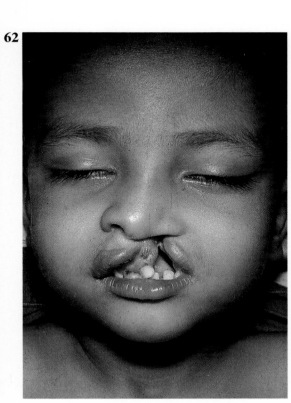

63

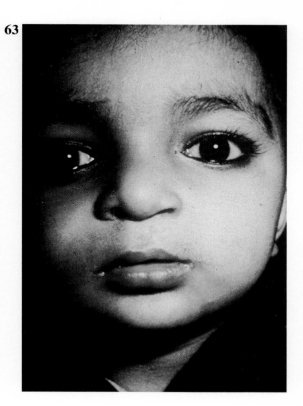

62 and **63 Left-sided unilateral cleft of complete type with marked alar flare and dropping alar margin.** Wide undermining of the lateral lip elements from the maxilla and in rolling of the alar margin produced a normal looking lip and a good Cupid's bow four years after the primary operation. May not require further touch up surgery.

64 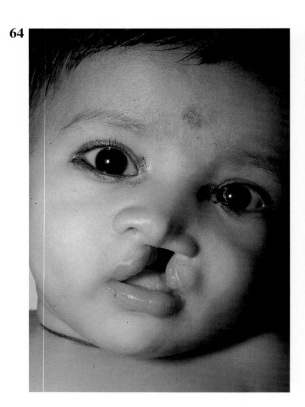 **65** 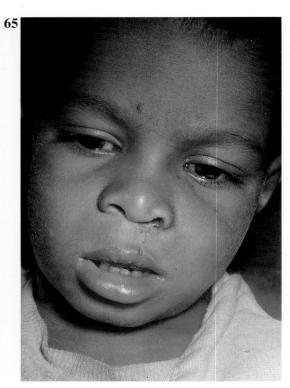 **66**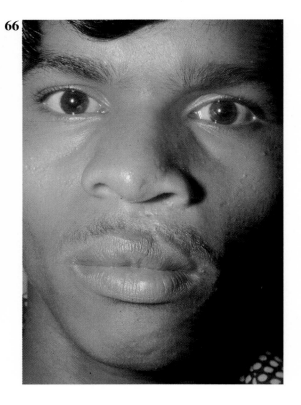

64 to **68**   **Left-sided complete cleft.** Regularly
followed up with touch-up surgery to the nasal
dome. Good job placement and well adjusted.
Alar rim excision will help.

67
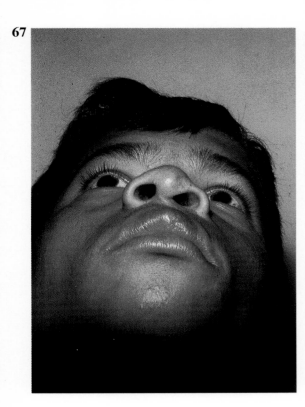

68
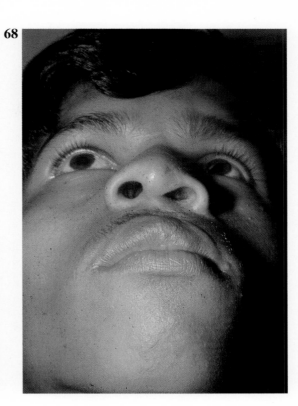

69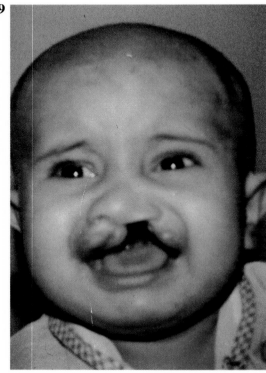

70

71

69 and **70** **A severe cleft with a wide maxillary gap and a difficult nasal deformity.** The actual body of the lip elements is reasonable. Radical rotation, columella lengthening, use of small amount of vestibule in lateral lip element advancement produced nasal symmetry and lip balance. The scar hypertrophy is improving gradually in this patient.

71 and **72** This case demonstrates several of the advantages of the R-A approach including an undulating Cupid's bow, an intact philtrum dimple, the natural position of the scar and the nasal correction. The effect of the tiny flap interdigitation at the mucocutaneous junction is particularly well demonstrated by the continuous 'white skin roll' which outlines the entire border of the upper lip without apparent interruption.

72

73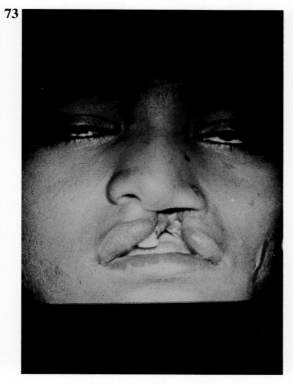

74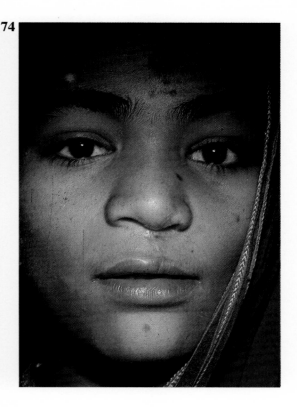

73 and **74** **Young girl of 15 with very wide complete cleft.** Radical rotation advancement produced good nose and good lip contour. Onlay graft to nose.

41

75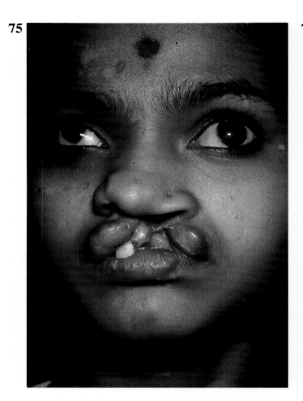

76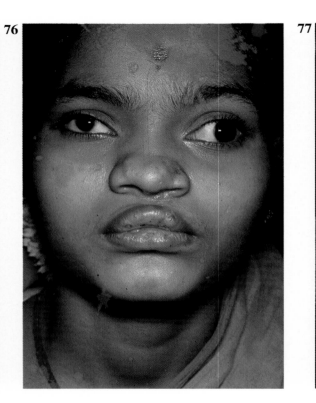

77

75 and **76   Young girl with wide cleft.** After radical R-A flap (**76**).

77 and **78   Nasal view in a primary incomplete cleft** showing widened nasal floor. Postoperative picture showing symmetrical nostrils.

78
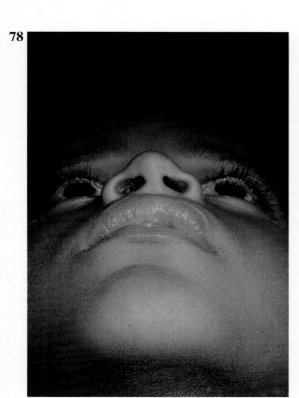

79
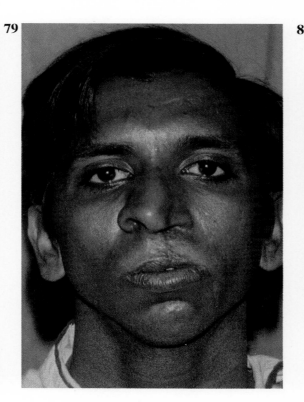

80
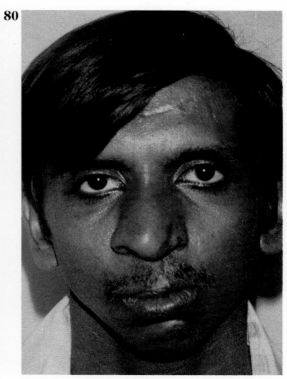

79 and **80** **Secondary cleft lip** in an adult operated elsewhere with marked deformity of the nose and a very poor scar line. Complete revision of the lip readjustment of alar base with a Z-plasty of the vestibular fold produced some visible change of the nasal contour. Patient satisfied with the cosmetic improvement in facial profile and now able to find employment.

81 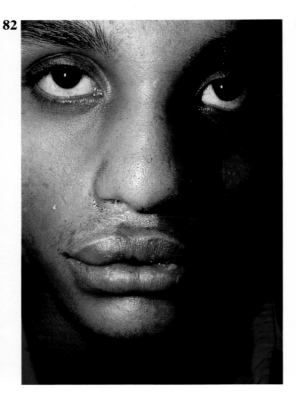 **82** **83**

81 and **82** **Unilateral cleft lip operated elsewhere** showing two common mistakes of a flared nostril-based and depressed groove in the lower mucosa. This could easily be due to poor approximation of the muscles as well as inversion of the mucosal stitches.

The whole lip repair was repeated to narrow the flared nostril and make it the same shape and size as the normal side. Note the good approximation of the mucosal layer.

83 **A secondary defect** in this girl who underwent surgery four times with a totally failed palate (not shown here) and grossly inadequate lip and nose defect. An artificial denture was necessary to start the process of repair. Complete revision of the lip repair and correction of nasal deformity by Joseph's incision.

Preventable deformities

1   Flared nostril floor. This is one of the most common deformities seen and is easily prevented in the primary operation. The distance between the two pillars of the alar on the normal side can easily be judged and the same distance kept on the affected side. The distance can even be shortened in the Millard operation by advancing the upper interdigitating triangles until the floor is exactly the same. In fact the author has found that a slight over-correction is in order to allow for a delayed flare in a couple of months. A flared nostril is one of the most common secondary deformities seen in practice. For its cure a quadrangular piece of tissue is removed and the floor equalised.

2   Poor suture line on the lip
   This may be due to various causes:

(A)   Approximation under tension.
(B)   Using too thick a suture material.
(C)   Tying the knot too tightly.
(D)   Keloid formation.
(E)   Depressed scar line.
(F)   Step deformity at the mucocutaneous junction.

There is no excuse for any of these mistakes except when unexpected Keloid forms. The step deformity is avoided by using the four dot method at the mucocutaneous junction line. Tying the knots too tightly reflects on the poor skill of the surgeon.

3   'Whistle' deformity of lower third of the lip. This is often due to poor muscle approximation and the giving way of the mucosal suture line due to injury or tension. The author prefers to use a vertical mattress suture at the mucosal level and good healing is the usual result. A tension relieving mattress stitch often helps for sound healing of this area when a wide cleft is closed.

4   Vistibular ridge inside the nostril. This is often due to the severe buckling of the middle of the lateral crus of the lower alar cartilage. It can be easily corrected by a combine Z-plasty of the mucosa cum cartilage. After this correction the external appearance of the alar depression markedly improves. This is often needed in secondary corrections.

5   Poor rotation of the Cupid's bow. A further rotation – advancement is needed to give a satisfactory result.

Secondary cleft lip

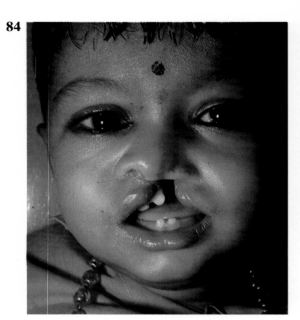

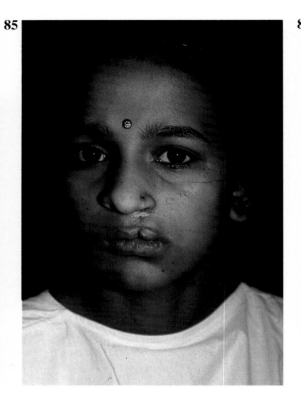

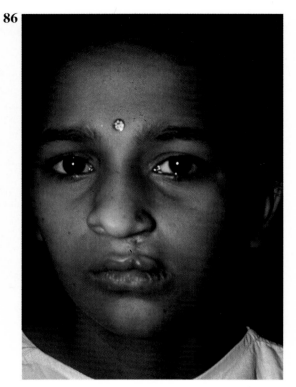

84   Baby Jain had a primary complete cleft lip of the left side which was operated in June 1962. Rotation advancement flap was used and the part healed without any problem. The child was three months old when surgery was performed.

85 and **86**   After 23 years, the same patient came for follow-up and showed secondary deformities:

1   Drooping of the nostril margin.
2   Flare of the floor of the nose.
3   A widened scar line.
4   A 'whistle' deformity of the lowest part of the lip. It was decided to operate on this case to correct all the four defects.

Operative steps

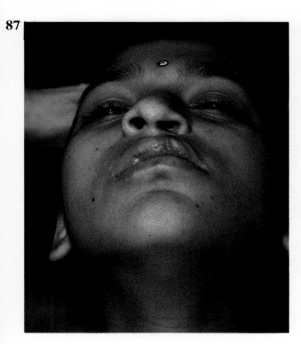

87 Nasal view of the same patient showing the widening of the floor of the nose as well as the notch in the lower part of the lip.

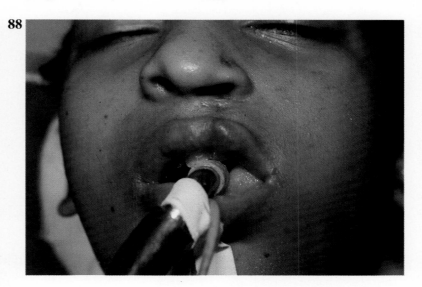

88 Patient is given general anaesthesia and intra-tracheal tube fixed on the middle of the lower lip. The throat is packed and the surgeon sits at the head of the patient.

89

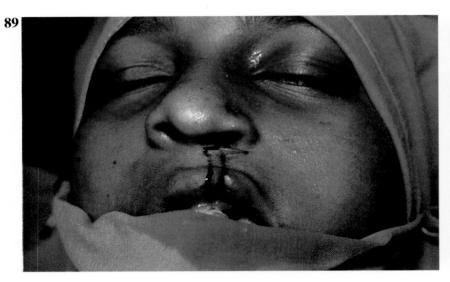

90

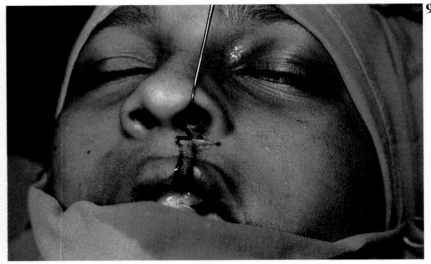

91

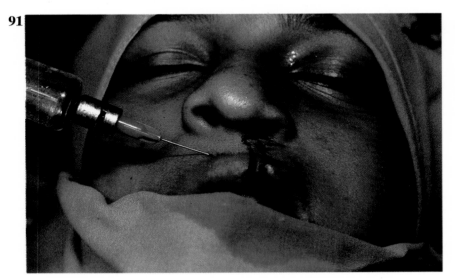

89   Double-line markings showing the stretched scar and the amount of narrowing to be done at the floor of the nose. The area of the 'whistle' defect has to be excised.

90   The roof of the nostril elevated by a skin hook showing the vestibular fold on the lateral side which will have to be corrected.

91   Medial segment of the lip infiltrated with saline-adrenaline solution.

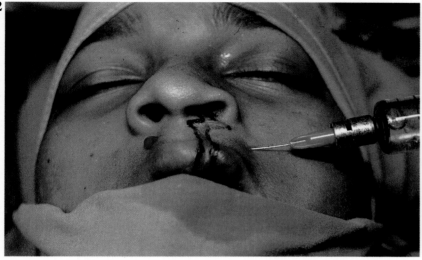

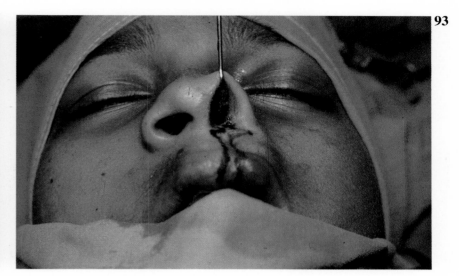

92 The lateral segment infiltrated in the same way. It is advisable to wait for a couple of minutes before starting the operation.

93 The vestibular fold area is identified.

94 The assistant compresses both the lateral and medial segments of the lip and stretches it downwards before the actual incision is started.

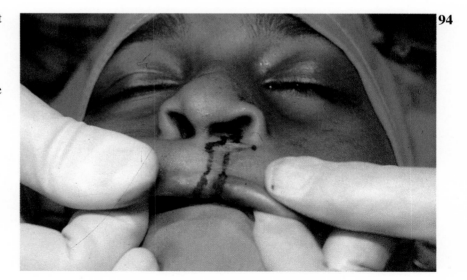

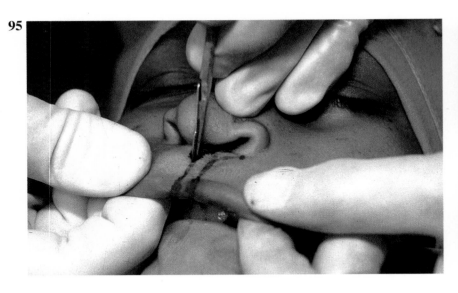

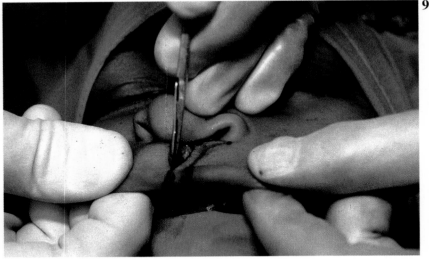

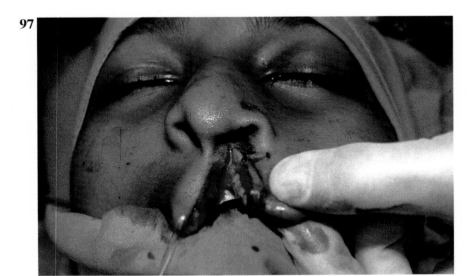

95 With a No. 11 Bard Parker knife, the medial incision is opened from above downwards.

96 The incision progressing in the lower segment of the lip.

97 The cut medial segment is held by a stitch and all the bleeding points are coagulated.

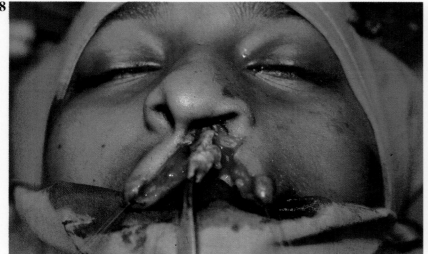

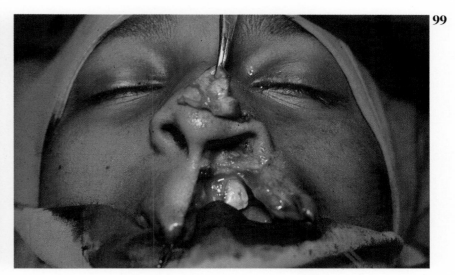

98 and **99**   A similar incision is made along the dotted line on the lateral segment extending from the floor of the nose to its lowest point. This flap is also held by a stitch. The redundant portion of the scarred skin muscle and mucosa are then dissected off and preserved in case it is needed later for an 'onlay' graft to raise the dome of the nose.

100   The vestibular fold is identified and infiltrated with saline-adrenaline solution.

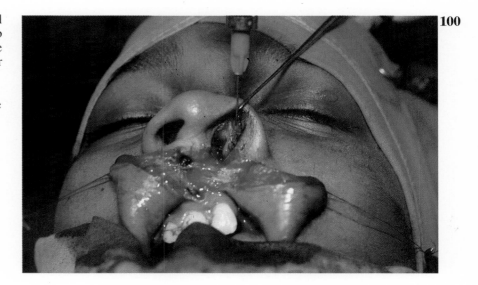

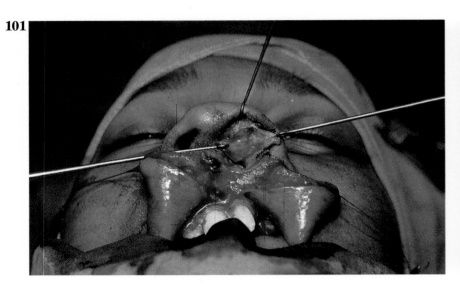

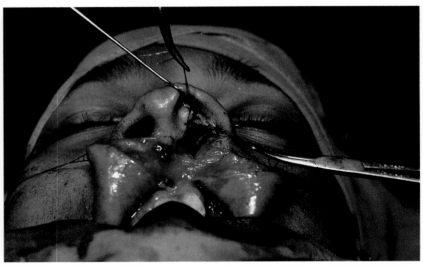

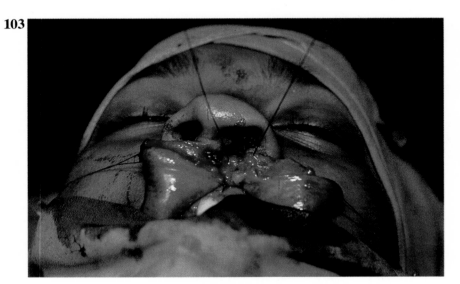

101   A Z-plasty is made at the vestibular fold and the flaps, including the mucosa and cartilage, are dissected from the skin surface. The two skin hooks are holding the Z-flaps.

102   The superior Z-plasty flap is transposed and held with a stitch and the inferior part is also stitched and held downwards.

103   The Z-plasty is already completed and the suturing of the muscular layer is started at the floor of the nostril using 3/0 Dexon. The knots are tied facing towards the mucosa and this helps in better healing of the skin surface.

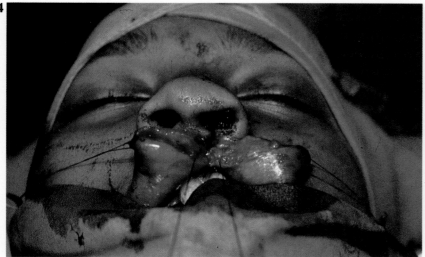

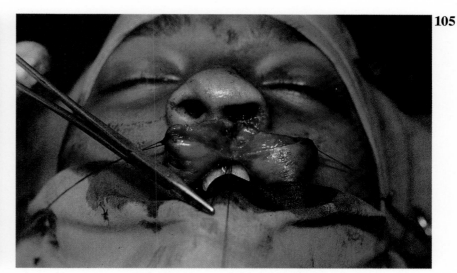

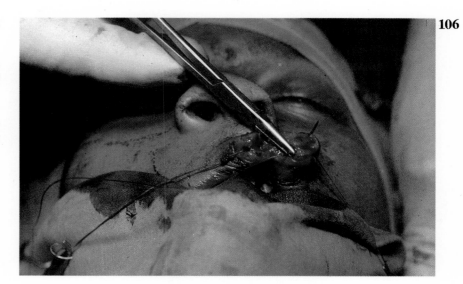

104 Suturing of the mucosal layer is commenced from above downwards using the same Dexon material.

105 The muscle closure is advanced. Notice that both floors of the nostril have become symmetrical. This is important as re-adjustment if necessary could be done at this stage.

106 The lowest muscle stitch through the lateral segment shows the amount of tissue that is picked up for good approximation and prevention of any 'whistle' defect.

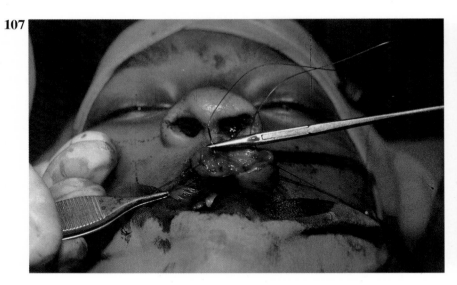

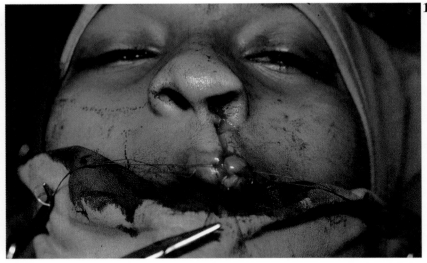

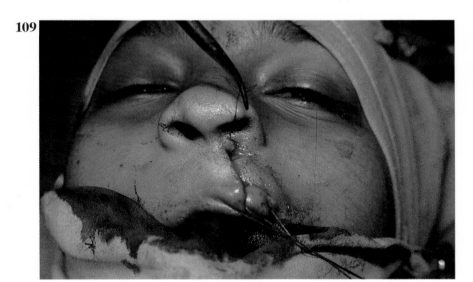

107 A similar stitch passed on the medial segment showing the knot which will be tied facing the mucosa or deep surface.

108 The skin margins automatically coming near to each other and showing the inter-digitating triangles at the floor of the nostril sill.

109 Closure of the uppermost part of the skin layers using 5/0 Prolene.

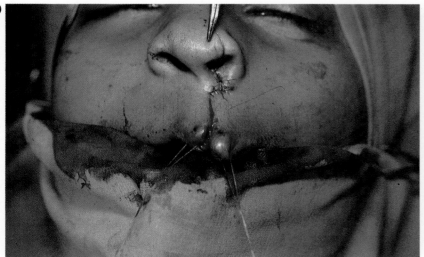

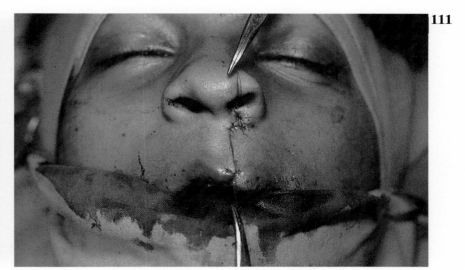

110   At the mucocutaneous level two more ink dots are added to facilitate the proper approximation of the mucocutaneous line.

111   The stitches holding the lower margin of the flaps are removed and the mucocutaneous points are approximated and held with an artery forcep.

112   The skin margins are closed with prolene suture. The knots are tied just snugly enough to prevent leaving stitch marks.

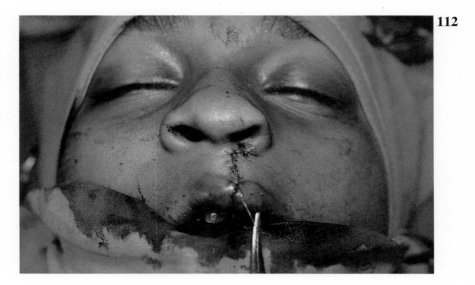

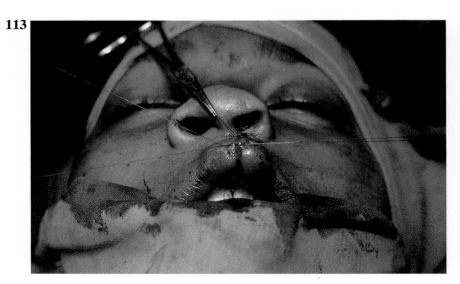

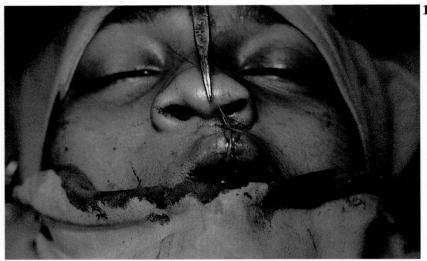

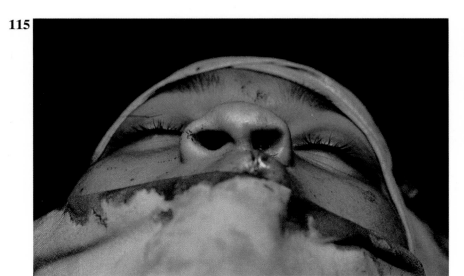

113 The mucocutaneous stitch is held up and the mucosal layer is closed by vertical mattress sutures. This is important in preventing any inversion of the mucosal layer.

114 Three vertical mattress sutures are made with Prolene. Notice the eversion of the mucosa.

115 Suturing is completed and it is noticed that there is an asymmetry on the cleft nostril side which will have to be corrected.

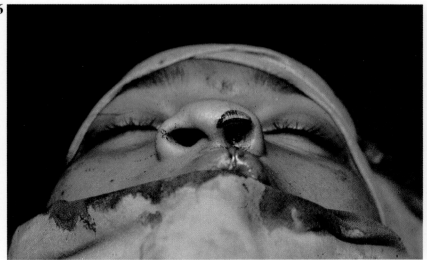

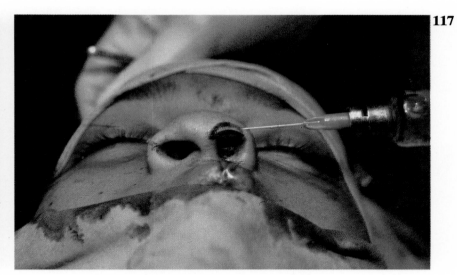

116 An ellipse of skin is marked at the site of redundancy.

117 The elliptical area is infiltrated.

118 The skin ellipse is excised and the surrounding skin margin is slightly undermined for better approximation.

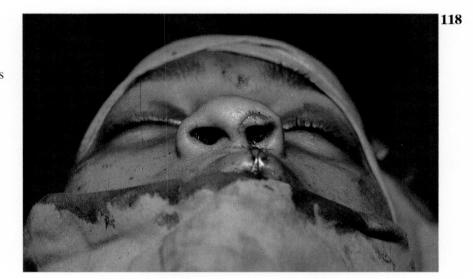

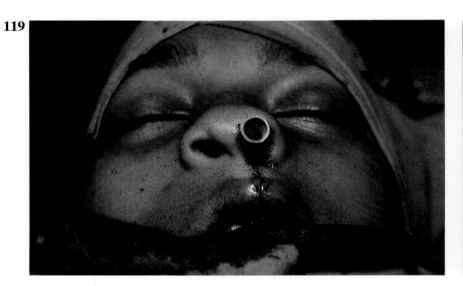

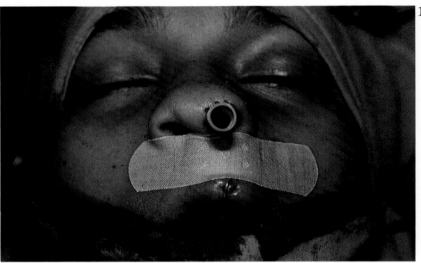

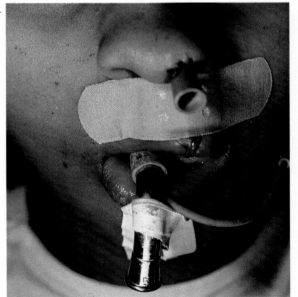

119 The elliptical defect is closed with 5/0 Prolene and a rubber tube inserted so as to compress the area where the Z-plasty has been performed. This tube is retained for 48 hours.

120 A surgical tape dressing is applied and retained for 48 hours. Notice the skin closure of the elliptical defect above the side where the tube is inserted.

121 Frontal view showing the intratracheal tube separated from the machine. Note the symmetry of the nose and the correction of the alar droop.

Conclusion

Present-day knowledge and techniques have not suddenly come into being, but have been built up from the cumulative observations of centuries, which have been passed on in literature. In 1362 Guy de Chaullac, the leading surgeon of the fourteenth century, completed a great textbook of surgery. In the prologue to this work he acknowledged the debt he owed to those who had gone before and he expressed his feelings in a picturesque way, 'We are like children standing on the shoulders of a giant, for we can see all that the giant can see, and a little bit more'.

My success in cleft lip surgery basically depends on two persons – Dr. Ralph Millard for such a monumental and excellent method of lip repair that more than half the plastic surgeons from all over the world have now adopted as the most ideal method, and secondly, to his mentor and father of plastic surgery, Sir Harold Gillies who first introduced me to this method in India and to whom I am most grateful. It is very well said of him:

In this century in which we are privileged to live and work, Sir Harold Gillies was one such giant of a man. Let us, metaphorically speaking, climb on to his shoulders, so that in the years that are yet to come, each of us who has students to teach, may be able to say to them with truth, and with pride in his voice, 'This man was one of my teachers'.

Many surgeons have discounted the importance of a method by saying that a surgeon should use whatever procedure he personally believes will work best for him. This attitude can lead to mediocrity. It is true that most experienced surgeons have their favourite lip method, and with this their results are better that with any other. Yet, no matter how skilled a surgeon may be, his best results are limited by the ultimate of the method he favours. A method's merit must be measured by the closeness of its approach to a natural looking and acting result. Cleft-lip surgeons must be perfectionists, free to aspire and willing to work in millimetres. If the method scraps the Cupid's bow, violates the dimple or allows the scar of the union to cross natural lines, then no matter how fastidious the surgeon is, he can never make up the handicap. There is, however, one essential factor which influences the outcome of any method. Before a technique can be made to attain its greatest potential, the surgeon must not only be familiar with it and believe in it, but actually woo it to its ultimate.

And finally the Millard operation has been practised since 1958 to give an opportunity to evaluate its advantages. The underlying principles are quite sound. It restores structures to their normal positions and hence a normal looking lip is the final outcome. Millard has aptly said 'a natural-looking result following closure of a congenital cleft is a work of art'. In fact it is a 3-D work of sculptured art. Principles, measurements, marks and incisions of a technique can be standardised and a blueprint of the technique memorised. Yet the last few millimetres which makes all the difference must depend upon the sculptor and his clay'.

All cleft lip cases require the finest surgery possible and if this is not provided in early childhood, the poor results will carry into the patient's life.

References

Berkeley W. T. (1959). The Cleft Lip Nose, *Plast. & Reconst. Surg.*, **23**, 567.

Braithwaite (1964). *Modern Trends in Plastic Surgery*, pp. 44.

Brauer, Cronin and Reaves (1962). Early maxillary Orthopedics, Orthodontia and Bone Grafting. *Plast. & Reconst. Surg.*, **29**, 625.

Burston W. (1960). The Presurgical Orthopoedic Correlation of Maxillary Deformity in Clefts of Both Primary & Secondary Palate, *Trans. Inter. Soc. Plast. Surg.* pp. 28–36.

Calnan J. S. (1953). Movements of the Soft Palate. *Brit. J. Plast. Surg.*, **5**, 286.

Cronn T. D. (1957). Surgery of the Double Cleft Lip and Protruding Premaxilla, *Plast. & Reconst. Surg.*, **19**, 389.

Davis A.D. (1951). Collective Review: Management of the Wide Unilateral Cleft Lip with Nostril Deformity, *Plast. & Reconst. Surg.*, **8**, 249.

Dorrance G. M. (1933). *The Operative Story of Cleft Palate*, Saunders Philadelphia.

Harkins C. S. (1958). Retropositioning of the Premaxilla with the Aid of an Expansion Prosthsesis, *Plast. & Reconst. Surg.*, **22**, 67.

Holdsworth W. G. (1957). *Cleft Lip and Palate*, Grune & Stratton, New York.

Johanson B. (1961). Bone Grafting and Dental Orthopoedics in Primary and Secondary Case of Cleft Lip and Palate. *Acta. Scand.*, **122**, 101.

Le Mesurier A. B. (1962). *Hare Lips and their Treatment*, William & Wilkins, Baltimore.

McIndoe A. and Rees T. D. (1959). Synchronous Repair of Secondary Deformities in Cleft Lip and Nose, *Plast. & Reconst. Surg.*, **24**, 150.

McGregor I.A. (1963). *Brit. J. Plast. Surg.*, **15**, 46.

Maneksha, R. J. (1956). *Plastic Surgery in the Tropics*, Popular Prakashan, Bombay.

Millard R. (1957). *A Primary Camouflage of the Unilateral Harelook*, *Trans of Inter. Soc. of Plast. Surg.*, 268 William & Wilkins, Baltimore.

— (1958). A Radical Rotation in Single Harelip, *Amer. J. Surg.*, **95**, 318.

— (1960). Complete Unilateral Clefts of the Lip, *Plast. & Reconst. Surg.*, **25**, 595.

— (1976) *Cleft Craft*, Part 1, Little, Brown & Co., Boston.

Nordin K. E. (1957). *Trans. Inter. Soc. Plast. Surg.*, pp. 228, William & Wilkins, Baltimore.

Oldfield M. C. and Tate G. T. (1964). Cleft Lip and Palate, *Brit. J. Plast. Surg.*, **17**, 1.

Peet E. (1961). The Oxford Technique of Cleft Palate Repair, *Plast. & Reconst. Surg.*, **28**, 282.

Randall P. (1964). *Modern Trends in Plastic Surgery*, pp. 17, 29.

Reidy J. P. (1958). 370 Personal Cases of Cleft Lip and Palate, *Ann. Roy. Coll. Surg. of Eng.*, **23**, 341.

— (1962). The Other 20 Per cent: Failures of Cleft Palate Repair, *Brit. J. Plast. Surg.*, **15**, 261.

Rehrmann A. (1964). *Modern Trend in Plastic Surgery*, pp. 50.

Schjelderup H. (1963). Late Correction of Severe Nasal Deformity in Unilateral Hare Lip Cases, *Acta Chir. Scand.*, **126**, 427.

Tempest M. N. (1958). Some Observation on Blood Loss in Hare Lip and Cleft Palate Surgery, *Brit. J. Plast. Surg.*, **11**, 34.

Veau V. (1931). *Division Palative*, Masson, Paris.

Index

Figures refer to page numbers